Coming
Through The
DARKNESS

Cancer and One Woman's
Journey To Wholeness

CLAUDETTE ANDERSON
COPELAND

Coming

Through The

DARKNESS

Cover Design By David Ferreira
Art & Design With A Positive Influence
of San Antonio, Texas

In Celebration of

All The Sisters

Who Have

Decided

To

Survive

And In Memory of the Ones Who Tried

CONTENTS

ACKNOWLEDGMENTS

I often muse at the paradox by which God has presented me into history. My script, concurrent with so many of my companions, has been that of "strong black woman"—teacher, preacher, sustainer. Yet the name my mother gave me, Claudette, means "little lame one." Perhaps she knew intuitively, of the woundings which are necessary to make women strong, and that in my lameness, God would *carry me* into an incredible destiny.

Special honor to my Mama, Edna Juanita Day, for your gentle beauty and for the lessons of unconditional love, and to my only "real" sister, Stacy Lynn Anderson Garner, whom I adore.

◇ To you Clara Mitchell, Executive Director of Destiny Ministries, for being my midwife and never leaving my side, as we birth 'destiny.' You saw what I did not. You are the absolute best!

◇ To my faithful Executive Assistant, Minister Denise Phenix Campbell, for your scrutiny, attention to detail and your standard of excellence, as we forged this manuscript, and everything else on my desk. Your covering prayers and wise counsel uphold me daily.

◇ To my circle of six, you know who you are to me. The preaching women mentioned in these pages who have been my refuge of friendship and prayer through the years. Jessica, Elaine, Joann, Cynthia, Renita and me. "Let's stay together."

◇ To my former assistant and unfailing friend, the Reverend Carolyn Ramsey-Allen, without whom I might have died. Thank you for holding my hand in the dark. Galatians 4:14.

◇ To my "Sweet Baby" Crystal Nicole, and Antonette. For awhile, the only family I had. You salved the wound that would not heal.

◇ To the faithful women of New Creation Christian Fellowship, San Antonio, Texas, past and present, for your love and honor throughout the years.

◇ To the hard working staff of Destiny Ministries: Bridgett McCarthy, Elizabeth Manuel, Irma Gunnels, Shirley Johnson, Quida Patterson, Nicole Harrell, Priscilla Bradford, Betsy Higgins and Jackie Saunders. My joy, my crown, my jewels.

◇ To Ben Simmons, Carl Booker & Avista Products. My jumpstart!

◇ Heartfelt gratitude to the Atlanta Connection: Heidi Lue, Kassan Bonner, Stephanie Tyson and Mr. Robert Ford of Majestic Media for the help you *are going to be.* The Washington Connection: Jeri Keyes and Mother Sylvia Turner. The Dallas Connection: Shewanda Riley and the Austin Connection: Sandra Ross. Philippians 1:3

◇ Humble appreciation to the volunteers who have given incredible ideas, leg work, gifts of time, talent and treasure as I taxi out onto the runway: Pastor Keith Graham, Cheryl Porter, Donna Perry, Arthur Sanderson, Linda Boykin, Deaconess Rosie Allen, Paula Barriner, Ramona Tipler, Deacon Darryl Marbury, Mary Holliday, James Bradford, Robert Tyler, Clifton and Jackie Johnson, Pauline Pitts, Michelle May, Beverly Pillot, Barbara Foster, Elaine Clark, Erica Lucas (Daughter of Destiny!); Jackie Saunders and Cynthia Ladison of the San Antonio Express News for your editorial insights, and Diane Hannah Jones for sacrificial late nights and the 'finest tooth comb', ever.

◇ To my special brother, David Ferreira, for the power of an image, and for the love that bathes the work you do for me, and for Christ. Thanks for pressing in.

◇ And to my beloved husband and friend, Bishop David Michael Copeland. Your "vision" has been the "hand at my back" pushing me to put this journey onto paper, and believing with me that someone would read it and be blessed. You helped me remember the details I missed. And later you helped me to forget the ones I couldn't. With you, I have weathered many dark nights and come full circle to points of Pure Light. 1 4 3.

INTRODUCTION

This book is not for everyone.

Some of you will find its contents contrary to your theology. You may accuse me of weakness or compromise because I openly acknowledge what some faith teachers deny: Suffering is an integral part of Christian growth. That is the story of the cross.

Others may be offended by the subject matter of personal suffering, death and dying. It is something you would rather not discuss, and certainly, you prefer not to spend money to read about it in a book.

Some of you will find portions too "preachy" and become bored with my attempts to share a Biblical understanding. Finally, others may shun the emotional realities, finding portions too "human" for your tastes.

But for the one person who is suffering, this little book may be for you.

If you are wondering "why?" or if you need companionship and comfort as you find your way through the darkness, may this book find its way into your hands. And if you love someone who is battling the physical and emotional ravages of life, perhaps these pages will offer you some guidance as to "how to be" in their midst. If you are preparing to soon meet the Lord, there are specific words from my heart, to you.

This is a cancer story. But it is more. It is the personal mapping that we all navigate on some level. Maybe your crooked convoluted journey is recovery from childhood victimization. Maybe yours is the rending of an unwanted divorce or burying your child; maybe it is losing your life's work through bankruptcy or fire or unexplainable treachery. Every person at some point, must find his or her way, swimming upstream in mud. This book is a story of feelings, thoughts and private reactions which may mirror your own while you are groping in the dark. It is to affirm that we are all more alike than we are different, and that we desperately need one another's kindness. No one makes it out of darkness alone.

Mostly it is a story of synthesis—how God uses the layers of life, to build a woman who will love Him. Here. And Hereafter.

I write to share a story of myself.

I write with you in mind.

I stand by the bed where a young woman lies, her face postoperative, her mouth twisted in palsy, clownish. A tiny twig of the facial nerve, the one to the muscles of her mouth, has been severed. She will be thus from now on. The surgeon had followed with religious fervor the curve of her flesh; I promise you that. Nevertheless, to remove the tumor in her cheek, I had cut the nerve.

Her young husband is in the room. He stands on the opposite side of the room, and together they seem to dwell in the evening lamplight, isolated from me, private. Who are they?, I ask myself, he and this wry-mouth I have made...Who gaze at and touch each other so generously, so greedily?

The young woman speaks.

"Will my mouth always be like this?" she asks.

"Yes," I say, "It will. It is because the nerve was cut."

She nods and is silent.

But the young man smiles.

"I like it," he says. "Its kind of cute."

All at once I know who he is. I understand and I lower my gaze. One is not bold in an encounter with a god. Unmindful, he bends to kiss her crooked mouth...I see how he twists his own lips to accommodate to hers, to show her that their kiss still works.

Richard Selzer, M.D.
From *MORTAL LESSONS,*
Notes on the Art of Surgery
(New York: Simon and Schuster, 1975) 45-46

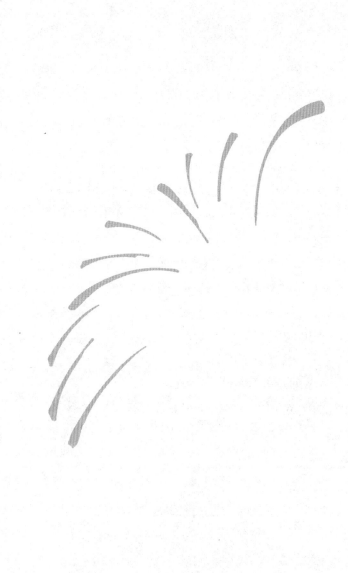

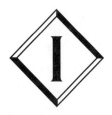

BIG GIRL FAITH

"My comfort in suffering is this:
Your promise preserves my life."
(Psalms 119:50 NIV)

I am a Christian. Saved. Sanctified. Filled with the Holy Spirit. I live right, love the saints, pay my bills on time, give abundantly, and play by the rules. I am a faithful wife, loyal friend, good citizen, and model church member. I color inside the lines. And none of it mattered.

I got cancer.

It was not supposed to happen to me.
But in the realm of faith, my great trial has been my great blessing.

Sometimes I wish I did *not* believe. I have written and re-written this "faith treatise", being jostled back and forth between personal integrity and theological correctness. I write first about faith, precisely because sometimes I wish I did not believe. For, once God has engraved God's outcomes on your life, one becomes a willing-or-not prisoner of this thing called faith. If I could dis-believe, or disentangle my soul from the constraining of this God – I could be free to kick and scream about my lot, to concoct schemes to compensate myself for my trouble, or to accuse God aloud in the assembly. I would be liberated to exact revenge upon my enemies instead of waiting on God; or I could simply turn and unceremoniously leave God. But alas, I do believe.

I believe the over-riding promise of Holy Scripture, even when the specifics elude me. I believe in the wisdom of the ages and the sages. I believe because the under girding memory of what God has done, keeps me coming back to Him in my heart, again and again, even when I think He is playing hide and seek with me. Faith is indeed a gift which I could never deserve.

In each decade of my life there are times I wonder if God has tricked me. Especially in the face of the awful contradictions in my experience. They keep mocking my faith and telling me to close my heart to the whole thing.

Daily I come to the very, very private pulpits of the counseling moment bearing witness to the dizzying pain, emotional torment, and unexplainable misery which people have been dealt. I find people desperate to still believe that God is alive. I ascend the public pulpit of the house of God knowing it is often despair which drives the masses to fill these pews. "Is there any word from the Lord?" I preach by the voice of God. I hear that sacred presence issue through my own clay lips. Sinners come to the altar of God, conquered and captured. The bound are set free. The sick are "hoped" and healed. The barely sane have their demons evicted. The tide of "faith which comes by hearing" sweeps up all who dare to stand in the path. I am good for God. Yet, superimposed upon these moments, *my life* grinds in miscellaneous pain. It is like the steel-upon-steel worn brakes in the raggedy car I used to drive. Unnerved. Flayed. Skinned alive. Mishandled to within an inch of my sanity. Life can be a hit-and-run experience, leaving you unable to get to your knees. Bloody, traumatized, clothing shredded and dirty, you grope for mercy in the middle of traffic. And the cars keep whizzing by, unable or unseeing or unconcerned about your survival.

But I keep getting up. And *you* will get up again, as well.

Sometimes I wish I did not believe, because it does not make sense to keep believing. But it is too late. Faith has organized my past and claimed my future.

In just a few days you too will encounter things you do not deserve, did not plan for, and will absolutely not believe are happening to you. The fact is "the same event happens to us all" (Ecclesiastes 2:14). But *how* you go through it, will build your character and help you discover that, in life, "the kiss can still work." Your trouble can nudge you, push you, shove you till your citizenship is in the high regions of faith!!

Mature faith is God's vehicle to land you at your life destination. It is a living, active, offensive weapon which God puts in your hands then teaches you to use by on-the-job training. It beams like a laser through the clutter of evil and demonic government. It exposes the 'god of this age' (II Corinthians 4:4) and gets you where you are going with all your "goods" intact. The renegade god operates in darkness and confusion, and refuses to relinquish his claim on humanity. Even on the redeemed. Mature faith guides you through the land mines he has buried in the terrain of your life. Despite the explosions you need not be ultimately destroyed!

• Real Life and Real Faith

Contemporary Christian doctrine expunges the role of "real life" in building your faith. Some teachers despise the very idea. They would have us believe that the only method of maturing in God is through the preaching, teaching, study and application of the Word of God.

I suggest to you that hearing preaching, teaching, study and even the personal application of the word are only pre-game practice. You never know whether you are growing in grace and sound in faith (fully persuaded, embracing, willing to die for the thing you have heard and studied) until you are obedient *in real life, under the hand of opposition or suffering.*

High spiritual principles—love, patience, longsuffering, gentleness, forgiveness—for example, usually stand in opposition to basic human nature. So does faith. They are not our first response. The higher your calling and assignment, the more stringent will be your training in spiritual life and godliness. Hence, you (your basic human nature) will always chafe under the discipline, and suffer *something* in order to line up with the higher plane. You will start off in a grossly imperfect family. You will sacrifice what you think you cannot live without. You will yield your rights. You will watch others have the apparent advantage. You will be slandered, misinterpreted, humiliated and not given the release to defend yourself. You will suffer in some way, in order to conform to the higher principles of spiritual life. You will be *trained in the classroom of suffering* to walk closely with God. The by-product will be a faith, which defies explanation, weds you to God's heart, and makes demons frantic—in real life.

Jesus, in His earth-walk "learned obedience" through the things that He suffered. There are extremely hard points in *our* lives, that seem absolutely senseless. The only option is to *learn* something! It is a high discipline to *willingly* follow Jesus there.

For hereunto were you called: because Christ also suffered for us. Leaving us an example that you should follow his steps. Who did no sin, neither was guile found in his mouth. Who...committed himself to Him who judges righteously. (I Peter 2: 21-23)

Suffering in real life exposes the guile, and the fleshly residue. You learn whether or not the spiritual ingredients of the Word, the Spirit and faith have actually been digested. Suffering whether private or public, inside or outside church walls, seeks to erode the very spiritual life which God is trying to develop. But rightly used, it proves, exercises and builds the muscle of faith. You will always confirm your faith, by obedience in the midst of suffering. Suffering stimulates the breast milk of faith, and brings it forth for your own survival.

Victory in suffering takes away the devils bullying tools. You will prove your worthiness for the assignments of spiritual life within the context of "real life." Both you, God and devils will know that you embrace what is right, noble and holy--by choice. Even as sickness and sorrow stand in your face, you resolve not to go the way of flesh. As my Mama used to admonish, you decide to "be a big girl." At every point, it is your decision.

"The way of flesh" is the tendency toward complaining, anger, bitterness, and accusing God. Its end is despair. It is the way that seeks *counterfeit comfort* because things are not going your way. It is the way of *secret indulgences and private rewards*, to soothe the hardness you are presently undergoing. It is the way *of retaliation and revenge*. And it is the spoiling of your heart.

For the son or daughter who resolves to grow up in the things of faith, and graduate from "faith to FAITH," suffering will turn into a blessing. Life, with its contradictions and losses will act as fertilizer to grow your faith. The "stinking stuff" will work into the soil of your life and, in the end yield fruit of staggering beauty.

• The Use of Suffering

I am not just speaking of suffering for suffering's sake. There is neither virtue nor reward in *simply suffering*. **Whenever possible, mentally healthy persons avoid relationships, escape individuals and alter circumstances which make us suffer**. Even when we allow for things which hurt us, *as a moral or ethical choice*, we do so from a position of spiritual strength, not from a mere need to demonstrate our victimization. We allow it for a long-range good, and a higher goal. Women particularly need reminding: taking abuse, becoming the willing victim and bewailing our perpetual martyrdom does not make us more holy or well loved. And it sometimes gets us killed or relegated to a prison or an asylum. In Original Purpose, our humanity and our person-hood must be honored at all times, as gifts from God. There must be a correct understanding and utilization of the seasons of suffering.

However, there arise events over which we have no control. With all our economic power, fasting and prayer, naming and claiming; with academic degrees and intellectual acumen; despite charm and beauty, holiness and virtue -- trouble lands squarely into our lives. In these moments we are boxed in by a reality which will not budge. We must enter the darkness, head on.

We have only one choice. "How, now, will I *use* this?"

This is an extremely difficult discipline. It must be prayerfully practiced, daily reinforced, and chosen over and over again in the spirit of your mind: *I will use these things which have hurt me, in order to build me.*

The correct use of suffering is the bridge that graduates us from a faith which is basic and elementary. Basic faith is foundational learning about God, the rudimentary principles of our salvation. This faith is the dependence on what we hear from week to week to sustain us. It is the meaning and essence of life in relationship to God. It is planted into your heart by what you hear.

Faith cometh by hearing, and hearing by the word of God. (Romans 10:17)

Depending on the condition of your heart/ soil, your life changes and you become a believer in Christ. Now you need "building" faith. Depending on the condition of your choices about hard things, your "substance" as a believer changes. Maturity begins.

Mature faith is the state of being fully persuaded about the *motives* of God. This faith is rooted in the goodness, the faithfulness, and the absolute love of God. It is not fragile and spindly faith, easily plucked up and blown over. It is "established" as the root system of a tree, through time and storms. Unshakable, unswerving, settled faith. This faith is born after having come through honest seasons of doubt. Weathering the apparent absence of God, and wrestling with my anger at God for deserting me, produces this quality of faith. Yet it is *the prize* for the person who stays with God until coming out on the other side. Its reward is a deepened understanding and a broader revelation of what God has in mind. *This faith takes the fear out of living and the terror out of dying.*

This is seldom a linear process. It is circuitous. It has many twists, turns and surprise detours. But once one has begun the journey, there is no option. You believe God for your future or you die like Lot's wife: stuck, frozen, fossilized in what might have been instead of what *can be*. Suffering—rightly used, undeserved, unplanned—will take you from faith which gets you *in*, to FAITH, which gets you *OVER*. However, there is no shortcut.

There are profound growing pains in reaching "big girl faith."

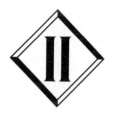

WHO IS GOD, TO YOU?

"I am not ashamed of the gospel of Christ...for therein is the righteousness of God revealed, from faith, to faith..."(Romans 1:16-17 KJV)

I am a preacher, by calling, by training and by profession. I am paid to speak on God's behalf. Some of you reading this are life-long, third and fourth generation Christians. Some are standing as outsiders, seekers, wondering if God really exists in light of all you have endured. Some are in full-time, professional Christian service. Others are students of the Church and its great preachers. We discuss God. We uphold the idea of God. We serve God. We live for God. But when pressed, <u>what</u> exactly, do we *believe* about *who God is* and how God acts in the world?

'Who God is,' is not solely the issue. Certainly, God is God, all by God's self, independent of us, apart from us, not needing the creation as proof of divine existence. That is settled theological fact.

But in your personal life, who God is, is only half of an incomplete discussion.

What do you really believe about God while you are suffering?

It will determine the outcome of difficult relationships which God may be using to mold your character. What is God's plan in this? It will determine your material blessings when you are lacking in finances, shelter, or the beautiful "extras" of life. Are they for you? How will you work for, wait for, use them or share them? What is God's mind about this? And it will greatly determine the quality and results of your relationship with God when you are sick and suffering. What is God's motive in allowing this?

Who is God, <u>and</u> <u>what</u> <u>do</u> <u>you</u> <u>believe</u> <u>about</u> <u>God</u> <u>when</u> <u>you</u> <u>are</u> "<u>going</u> <u>through?</u>" Faith determines follow through.

• The Nature of God

The righteousness <u>nature</u> of God is brought to light by "what we preach," when we really preach the gospel. *(Romans 1:17-18)* It is what makes the gospel "good news" and not merely "news." Much contemporary preaching is simply frustrated ventilation introduced by a scripture. It is often ego-driven rhetoric which seeks to put people down, prove a point, control behaviors or punish adversaries in the pew. It may be "preaching" but little of it is good news.

The good news is that God has triumphed for us, in Christ, and always leads us in triumph! Despite the deteriorating, destructive, alienated state of His creation, God's kindness and mercy override it all. He raised Jesus, and does again and again in us, what He did in His Son. But isn't it a difficult thing, humanly speaking, NOT to be suspicious of God? God is experienced in the way our disappointing parents treated us: prone to abandon, certain to whip, often to withhold the privileges we thought we deserved. If you are a thinking person, you consider the worldwide plight of humanity. Hunger, plagues

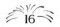

and diseases like AIDS; war, violence, homelessness, and secret horrors against vulnerable little children make God seem at best, like an absentee landlord or a powerless power. It would be "natural" to let the earthly shape our image of the heavenly. It seems difficult to be convinced about the merciful, healing and restoring nature of a God who has left so much to go wrong in the earth. And yes, sometimes, in our own personal lives.

• Is God Like Me?

Our experience of humanity often shapes our image of the Divine. Especially our own personal "humanity." Even as Christians. You know you. I know me.

When ignored, we ignore—or demand our right to attention.

When betrayed, we–if only unconsciously–entertain ways to get even.

When we are injured, or wounded, we fight back or withdraw.

When people fall short of our standards, we leave them to their own consequences.

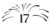

The fallen nature easily reverts to pettiness and payback. The preservation of "self" usually wins over love for others.

On some level, we believe that God is like us. We are seldom gracious and forgiving to those who fail to meet our own personal requirements. We forgive little. We remember much. Seldom do we go out of our way to rescue another. We are not like God.

My husband and I have a friend, Brother Saul, who is the number one sales representative in a major nationally recognized insurance company. He has, for several years, held this distinction and is honored worldwide for his accomplishments, which have netted the company multiplied thousands. A friend of Saul's had procrastinated and ignored his own insurance needs for years. Then his friend was stricken with cancer. Because of this pre-existing condition he was now uninsurable. When Saul found out, he went to the president of his company and said this: "If there is any favor on my life with this company, take it off me and give it to my friend. Allow me to write him a policy." The president refused. It had never been done. It could not be done. He repeated and was denied. A third appeal was made. "If there is any favor on my life with this company, take it off me and give it to this man." The president did what had not been done. He bound the policy. Not only for the sick man's life, but to insure the future of his wife, his children and his children's children. The favor was taken off one man's life, to redeem another.

God is like that.

Through the gospel we understand that God has not the same nature as humans. We have fallen short of God's standards, short of deserving God's love and favor. He takes the favor that was placed on his Son, and puts it on undeserving people. He "creates" good out of our apparent failure. God has not paid us back for our sins although we have procrastinated, and ignored Divine requirements. God makes peace with us, through His son Jesus Christ. He writes the policy. *And He himself* pays the premium. God, *thank God*, is not like us.

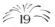

- **God and Payback**

> *What has happened to us is a result of our
> evil deeds and our own great guilt; and
> yet our God, you have punished us less
> than our sins deserved. (Ezra 9:13 NIV)*

Under the New Covenant, sickness, loss,
bereavement, and life's reversals are not,
generally speaking, divine retribution for our
ways. Yes, sometimes there are correlating
consequences. Cause and effect. Action and
results. Reaping and sowing are a part of
natural and supernatural law. If I smoke for
30 years, then become a Christian and stop,
there is a natural law that has been put into
motion, and may yield consequences of lung
cancer. If I have neglected my mate, cheated,
been emotionally and sexually unfaithful, even
though I "get right with God," laws have been
set in motion in the realm of human
relationship. He or she may leave me. If I have
failed to make choices in my youth about goal
setting, education, earning and saving money
or planning for my future, there are certain
probabilities that I will arrive at middle age in
a condition of "lack." *None of these conditions
and consequences should be interpreted as*

the actions and retributions of a God who is against you. The consequences are the result of our own human ignorance and bad decisions. Sin itself has its own penalty. That is why God sets boundaries to keep us from it.

Nonetheless, God is at work in every action, to bring His overall purpose to pass. Believe this and shape the results you expect and receive in the realm of faith. Unless we anchor in this faith stance, we will interpret all of life as the *meanness and judgement* of God and miss the loving purpose.

Perfect (mature) love drives out all fear, for fear has to do with [the expectation of] punishment and torment. (1 John 4:18 paraphrased)

There is a place of manifested potential, acquisition of good things, reconciliation in broken relationships, and recovery from disease. Bring your understanding of God into line with the Gospel – Good News. You will never expect that God wants to bless your life in "good measure" if you believe in a God who is always poised to clobber you.

I linger on this foundation because many who read this, are struggling against the "accuser." You are expecting payback. You think you are living under divine retribution. You may have AIDS because of your former lifestyle. You may be childless or infertile because of past abortions or poor sexual choices. You may have suffered a divorce and lost your children because you were not a faithful partner or a good parent. You may have suffered great financial losses in your home, or your business. Perhaps you have been publicly disgraced because of moral failures in your ministry. **And in your suffering, while you are down, the enemy, people and your own thoughts are ganging up against you!!** Your mind is telling you that God is "out to get you." Condemnation and fear are separating you from your legal right to forgiveness and acceptance, by faith. If God marked our iniquities, who could stand?

The Old Covenant rested on the legal requirements of God: upon violations of men, and the vengeance of God. It is written, "An eye for an eye, and a tooth for a tooth." The Old Covenant emphasized righteousness by works and penalty for failure. Repentance and forgiveness were echoed themes, having to be reinstituted with every ritual. Now Jesus Christ satisfies all debts, pays the penalties due and makes peace with the Father for us. We enjoy the kindness and the mercies of God, "with no condemnation." *(Romans 8:1)*. Penalty and punishment come only because we refuse to seek and obtain forgiveness. Forgiveness is the first order. He has punished us far less than our sins deserved, erased our records, then declared us "not guilty."

> *He who spared not his own son, but delivered Him up for us all, how shall He not with Him, also freely give us all things? Who shall lay anything to the charge of God's elect? It is God that justifies. (Romans 8:32-33 KJV)*

Have you earnestly repented? The accuser must shut his mouth. God is <u>not</u> out to get you.

You are justified.

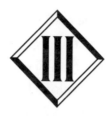

SEALED ORDERS

"Why is light given to a man, whose way is hidden?" (Job 3:23 NKJV)

God gives us memory. He allows us to look out of the back door of our lives, and reflect on where we have been. Hopefully we learn, and are made wise.

But God in His mercy, seals off the front door of our lives and forbids us to see what lies ahead. We would rush to it prematurely. Or we would fear to go. Maybe that is what the "walk by faith" is really all about.

In bringing you to mature faith, deep pure character, and in solidifying your relationship with Him, God seldom reveals the path you will take. He causes you to love Him first. He speaks deeply to your life, fills you with Himself, and drenches you with the joy of knowing Him in the pardon and freedom from sin. He gives you a honeymoon, in a season not unlike a new marriage. He is building emotional and worshipful intimacy with you. God is nursing you, speaking often and near to you, teaching you to walk with Him as His precious child. You find your joy on the lap of God, and at the milk of God's breast.

But you must mature. And He never tells you what the costs are.

If He did, you would never want to grow up.

He brings you into the family of God with "sealed orders."

• I Said I Would Go

I served in the United States Air Force as a military officer. As such, I was a "woman *in* authority, and under authority." Men and women under my authority were sworn to obey all lawful orders. I was likewise sworn to protect, obey and defend the Constitution and all that pertained thereto. I lived my life under orders. Orders and regulations governed the minute details of my life: the uniform I wore daily, where and when I reported to work, and even where in this world I would live, and possibly, die. When I was commissioned, I was saying to those in authority over me "I will go." The specific destinations had never been discussed.

At certain levels of service there were those who received assignments or "orders" to regions that were not publicly known. One might inquire of them, "Where will you be stationed?" and the reply might be, "In Egypt." But the specific whereabouts *in Egypt* were not divulged, because they had not been made known; not even to the airman or the soldier. The orders were, as it were, "sealed" until he or she was en route, on the plane, over the water.

There are some specifics about your destination, which God does not reveal, even to you, until you are "on the plane, headed for the site." Then God says, "Now you can open the sealed envelope and read the fine print." If you had known the specifics beforehand, you would not have said "yes."

If you had known the fine print you would have discussed it with your friends, and they would have talked you out of the journey. You would have shared it with your family and they would have tried to accompany you. Some places in God you must come alone.

In your "Yes Lord," you were handed sealed orders. You said, "I will go." Now you see. "These" are the steps to your perfection in Christ. "This" is the way to your holiness. "That" is the season of suffering waiting to purify your character. The unimaginable may be the very thing, which purges your old fleshly, selfish and superficial ways. You are on board now. The future is unknown, uncharted, and you have not been this way before. But you said you would go.

You will have to trust the motive of the commander.

• Revealing Christ

You go into your future with orders. You, as His ambassador, shall represent Jesus. The territory will be alien and hostile. Barriers high. He will have only one entrance into His estranged world. That entrance is *inside you*.

> *Always bearing about in the body the dying*
> *[agonizing suffering] of the Lord, that the*
> *Life of Christ may be manifest [revealed]*
> *in our mortal body...and since we have the*
> *same spirit of faith... He who raised up the*
> *Lord Jesus will also raise us up.*
> *(II Corinthians 4:10,13,14 NKJV)*

In the midst of this journey into unknown regions of suffering, dark murky waters and uncharted territory, God has an over-riding purpose: The *you that was seen* becomes the *Christ that is known*. In flesh, ambition, in intellectual striving and worldly preoccupation, spirituality is often extremely obscure. In your fatness and safety, Christ's life is so faint, so inconsistent. God must find a way to get that Life which he invested in you, at conversion, to become a *life force*, which makes a difference in this present world. Something in you must die, so that something of Him can live.

There is no other evidence that we belong to God, but that we reveal our resemblance to God as sons and daughters, right here in the earth-realm. The creation groans, awaiting manifestation of the children of God! Where are we? Who are we? We could have been taken out of the world at the moment of conversion, to be with God immediately. But we are left here on the earth, for the long range good. We are here to bear the image of the One who lives inside us.

> *We have this treasure in earthen vessels (clay jars), that the excellence of the power may be of God and not of us...*
> *(II Corinthians 4:7 KJV)*

But what happens when Christ's beauty and excellence are obscured by the vessel in which He lives?

God works from the inside out, by the Word engrafted, the Blood applied and the Holy Spirit given.

God also works from the outside in. Sometimes that work is through allowing affliction. It can act as a chisel. It chips. It conforms. It reveals.

God must excavate. He must allow life to "dig inside you." He must allow some seasons where you marinate like meat in circumstances you did not choose. God will soften the hard exterior. There is a living nugget of Himself you have hidden away, underneath your rights, your pleasures and your flesh nature. God will raise up "the Jesus in you." God will reduce the "you" which obscures Jesus.

This light affliction which endures for a moment works for us a far more exceeding and eternal weight of glory. (II Corinthians 4:17 KJV)

The season of affliction works for us by working *on us*. It "wears away" something within the earthen vessel. When the soul or the body are processed in suffering, the radiance of the Holy Spirit treasure becomes apparent. Natural priorities become worn as a loose garment. We care less for the things of this life. (This is why people who have been processed can be trusted <u>with</u> things of this life.) Christ shows Himself in our conversation, our temperament, and our compassion. Our outlook on life is transformed concerning things here, and hereafter. After rightly discerning the lessons of affliction, we "reveal Christ" most purely.

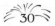

It is good for me that I have been afflicted that I might learn Thy statutes.
(Psalm 119:71 KJV)

Digest this! Believe this! Let this truth organize your perspective on all things. Then in days of sickness, reversals, or suffering, you can go from faith to FAITH. You can utilize the hard, hard days, as schoolmasters who will tutor you in obedience and discipline. Faith in God's motive will harness your thought life, tame your unruly tongue, and melt your apathetic heart. You'll know your suffering is carving out a place inside you for God's dwelling, *in such capacity that you have never known.* Large Christians have undergone large pain. Major prophets, major affliction. It opens a place in the heart for Him.

It is worth it all to reveal Christ to those who cannot see Him, except in you.

These are your orders, and they are mine.

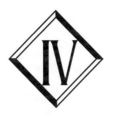

BASIC TRAINING

*"But do not say 'I am only a child.' You
must go to every one I send you and say
whatever I command you. Do not be afraid
of them..." (Jeremiah 1:7-8a NRS)*

The Lord began to deal with me at ten years
of age.

God placed a hunger inside me for Himself,
which I did not understand. No one in my family
could recognize or explain it. So I attached
myself to people in my neighborhood who took
me to their churches and honored my spiritual
curiosities. People who evangelize lost children,
know not the destinies they are salvaging. I will
always thank God for Mrs. Juanita Williams who
lived across from us, and Mrs. Viola Nesbitt who
lived up the street. They whetted my appetite
for the atmosphere of God's house. I humbly
appreciate my dear Mother who taught me the
little she knew, and first taught me how to pray.

I sat in Baptist churches, enthralled by the mosaic stained glass and the strong dignified deacons who executed the rituals of prayer in a fugue of word and chant. I sat in Methodist churches, enchanted by the complex five-verse hymnody, whose words made my heart yearn to know the writers, long ago dead. I sat in Holiness churches where I discovered the real presence of God amid the painted-by-hand shabbiness of the store front church. There God was, the High and Holy One, juxtaposed against the informality of a well-lived-in house. I wandered into Catholic Vacation Bible school where the fine brocade on the altar of the high church, and the smells of incense transported me to a place far beyond my pre-teen understanding. The austere black habits of the nuns made me wonder-fleetingly-if *I* would one day be cut out for the convent. I got on my knees, longing for what *I now know* was the true and living God. At eleven, I caught the bus alone to go to "tent meetings" which the sanctified church held in the neighborhood, and watched a lady preach the Gospel. The word, the scene, the fervor engraved itself upon my soul. Twenty years later I would meet and serve with that same lady, Dr. Ernestine Cleveland Reems of Center of Hope Church, Oakland, California. God made small, permanent deposits inside my spirit, which little by little were claiming me for Himself.

Immediately after the word is sown into the heart, the enemy comes to steal it before it can be established. (Matthew 13:19) I was drowning in unrecognized grief. May the hearts of parents be softened to the terrible chaos your teenagers may be battling, sitting right under your own roof. My parents had just divorced. I was grieving the absence of my beloved Daddy. I was trying to fit in with a new stepfather who seemed to despise my presence, and a mother who was working all the time, preoccupied with trying to hold a family together. I was angry and disappointed with everyone who mattered so I took it out on those who did not matter. In the girl gangs I was fighting at school every week. I was severely depressed, using alcohol and marijuana, and sitting alone in my room much of the time. Any given evening I was smoking a joint, blowing smoke out the window — and reading my Bible with a veil of sin over my mind.

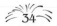
But I was drawn continually to the local gospel radio station. Dr. Mattie Moss Clark and the Southwest Michigan State Choir, would sing "Salvation Is Free." I longed to know, *What is salvation? And could it be for me? Where could I find this God?*

Crying out. Grieving. Seeking. I needed God. If you want to be right, God will not let you be wrong. Though the journey takes long stretches and winding turns, the heart that seeks will always be led to God. God arranges the encounter personally.

- **Sustained for a Future**

  The spirit of a woman sustains her in her infirmity but a wounded spirit who can bear? (Proverbs 18:14 paraphrased)

The year was bleak. Yet my emotional suffering was being used to put a "seek" in my soul, and would ultimately lead me to a saving relationship with Jesus Christ.

That year I contracted active Tuberculosis. Thirteen years old. I was taken to the doctor one evening, and rushed immediately to the hospital and into surgery. Surgeons operated on my collapsed lung, and for weeks drained the fluids from my thoracic cavity through tubes as large as garden hoses. My spirit was dying. It was too weak and wounded to sustain my body. I was kept out of school for a year by the health department, and had a tutor from the school board assigned to teach me. I was cut off from my classmates. My baby sister had been sent "down south" to my grandmother. The only person I had to love was now, gone too. I was sad all the time. I was cut off from my daddy. Cut off from my mother and stepfather, though they were in the house. Cut off because anger, withdrawal and a strong spirit of rejection were trying to own me and cancel my destiny.

Even as a child, I sensed that God must separate those whom He will use. There are public people, adored and admired, who affect crowds in great churches and crowded coliseums. They are exalted in the media and in the marketplace. There are icons who contribute in broad political arenas; others provide transforming social service to the masses – the Mother Theresas of the world.

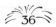

Yet I suspect that they all live their "real lives," their genuine lives in small private spaces with God. I learned the value of *running hard into God*, in the midst of isolation. God was sustaining me for a future I could never have envisioned. God tutored me to seek His presence, to find comfort in His nearness, and to value the companionship of the Almighty above human companions and crowds. Yet I had one friend, Mary Lou Lewis, who was faithful and consistent in seeking my soul. (She is currently the First Lady of Union Temple Baptist Church, Washington, D.C.) She *kept* on telling me about Christ. I was just thirteen years old when I heard the plan of salvation and my spirit stood at attention. Destiny situated me in the cleavage between suffering and the salvation message. The Lord marvelously saved my soul, and my life.

• Try Me Now and See

While convalescing at home, the doctors prescribed a regiment of twenty-four pills every day to treat my disease. After a season of treatment, though I could not return to school, I was no longer contagious and was allowed to venture out into public arenas. My friend Mary invited me one Friday evening to a small Church of God in Christ. Elder Urise Chillis was the pastor who called that night for those who would believe God by faith for their healing, and I was one.

> *Is there any sick among you? Let him call for the elders of the church; and let them pray over him, anointing him with oil in the name of the Lord: And the prayer of faith shall save the sick, and the Lord shall raise him up; and if he has committed sins, they shall be forgiven him. (James 5:14-15 KJV)*

The preacher laid his hands on me. For the first time in months, I felt a literal weight lift off my chest! It was as if God rolled something off my life, and I felt it manifest in a specific locality in my body. The world will never know what miracles are wrought in modest circumstances and out-of-the-way places, for little people who earnestly seek the Lord.

The next week was one of amazement and agony. I knew I was healed. I knew it in my thirteen-year-old soul. Yet I had a Mama who knew little about this God, and who was suspicious of the ways of these "sanctified people." Furthermore, I was still under a medical mandate – 24 pills every 24 hours. But in my soul I kept hearing, "Try Me now, and see." Without telling her, I stopped taking my medication, knowing that I had an appointment with the doctors at the health department the following Friday. If they said I was still sick, I would go back on my medicine and no one would know the difference. But I *knew* I was healed. I was treading in water I had never been in before. And the water was murky. What if? What if not?

I hasten to add that I am not a medical doctor. For the reader who is hanging in the balance, I do not advocate taking yourself off prescribed medication. God works through medicine just as He works supernatural miracles. (If God was not at work, even the medicines could do you no good!) When God has actually performed the healing, the doctors will confirm it. Then the medicines will work against the natural function of a healed body.

• A Voice Behind Me

The next Friday, I caught the bus as usual to the Erie County Health Department, Buffalo, New York. It was housed in the basement of City Hall. I had my baby sister back home with me, and it was my job to care for her while my Mama worked. I was called in as usual for my X-ray; seated, as usual, until the X-ray was developed.

Then came the nurse with a large paper sack containing my thirty-day supply of medication – as usual. My heart sank. I was stunned. I mechanically took the medication and started for home. Walking up the steps from the health department basement offices, I headed toward the bus stop. The ground was blurred by my tears. A 2-year old baby sister tagging along at one hand, medicine sack in the other. I was devastated.

I was thirteen years old, and I was depending on God.

Unexpectedly, I heard a voice behind me. That same nurse, with squeaking shoes ran to catch me, calling, "Miss Anderson, Oh, Miss Anderson! You will need to come back. Something is wrong with your x-rays!!" God was about to take me from faith, to FAITH. Sometimes you cry as you walk into a future that seems devoid of the activity of God. But the experience is already behind you; it was secured "in the spirit realm" when you prayed, believing. The guarantee is already delivered. God has done the work, and it will not be hidden for long. The voice will speak out, signifying that you have been with God!

I was invited back into a room with two doctors…a little black girl with her baby sister, and the invisible God, my personal physician. One of the physicians was seated at a desk. One walked back and forth before the lighted X-rays on the wall. He scratched a pink bald spot on his head with a pencil eraser. The pacing one began to explain to me what he saw. The pictures from the previous month, he pointed out, showed the shrunken, diseased lobes of my lung. And likewise, those from the month before.

But something was dramatically different on the pictures today. He did not see what he had seen before. When I asked him what it meant, all he said was, "I don't know, but you do not have to take that medication any more. We are prepared to release you today."

Now no chastening [discipline] seems to be joyful for the present, but grievous; nevertheless afterward it yields the peaceable fruit of righteousness to those who have been <u>trained by it.</u> (Hebrews 12:11 NKJV)

Suffering can be a training ground for faith in God! There is the point, an intersection, a breaking through where your trouble bows down, and hands over a payoff to your faith. Faith is the present possession of favor even before you get the goods! It is *grace, right now* to live joyfully while you're waiting. Faith now, extends *hope* into your future. The Old Testament word for 'hope', Tiquah in its original meaning, is "stretched tight as a rope." Faith <u>now,</u> extends hope like a life-line into your future. We keep pulling ourselves *through suffering* toward the promise of God. Sometimes that lifeline is as

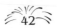

tenuous as a "tightrope" and you walk into your future with careful, well-placed steps. But faith *now,* gives us hope for then. So we keep putting one foot in front of the other.

Over thirty years later, each time I have a physical examination, doctors inquire about the foot long surgical scar around my rib cage and the residual shadow on the X-rays of my right lung. There is evidence of the trouble I had. It is always a witness that God was bigger than that season. God's love was greater than that trouble. My scars are His signature on my body, as my Redeemer.

I was thirteen years old. God had just given me my first course in *basic training*.

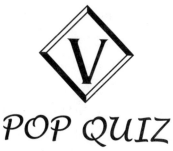

POP QUIZ

"Behold, it is planted. Now will it thrive...?"
(Ezekiel 17:10 NKJV)

What you hear preached on Sunday, you will be quizzed on by Wednesday.

What you think you have learned today, you will be tested on tomorrow.

What you have secured by faith yesterday, the devil will come to challenge today.

What you have mastered this year will need updating next year.

And God does not always announce the testing beforehand.

I got settled into a church home where I was encouraged, exercised and utilized for Jesus Christ. I returned to high school. I became a cheerleader, student government leader and an all around young Christian. I was bold and unapologetic in my witness, and yet grounded in being a teenager. I was the "young missionary" on an upward march in ministry, Bible in one hand, tambourine in the other. Hallelujah!!

Thank God I was in a good church home and under a wise Pastor, Bishop LeRoy Anderson of the Prince of Peace Temple, Church of God in Christ. Our leaders did not strip young people of their natural youth inclinations. Youth who are forced to submerge the normal adolescent curiosities, activities and developmental stages, usually boomerang. They find themselves in their twenties, thirties and even in mid-life, trying to recapture what "the church" did not allow them to experience when they should have. Our leaders guided us in holiness as we learned to negotiate our way in the world. It had been a good year.

But one morning at the age of fourteen, I awakened with such excruciating pain and fever that I could hardly walk. I was hospitalized again. Was it sickle cell anemia, a new disease they were discovering among people of color? Was it all in my mind? Attention-getting behavior? Or maybe covert child abuse, the psychiatrist and social worker inquired? Migratory juvenile rheumatoid arthritis was the verdict. An auto-immune disease; the body turns on itself and literally destroys the joints. I was in unimaginable pain. Deep pain. Radiating pain. Pain that took away my concentration. Pain which ushered in a fear of growing up. Fear of again having to be supported by drugs and chemicals. Fear. "Get her ready for physical deformities, a compromised lifestyle, and eventually a wheelchair. There is no cure."

Pain makes cowards of us all.

But I had already passed "basic training" just last year. That was a "lion." This was a "bear."

As soon as I was released from the Deaconess Hospital, I purposed to make my way to the House of God.

• Run For Cover

Whenever you are in prolonged seasons of suffering, there are times when you will not want to be "bothered" with people. You may battle anger and resentment about your condition. You will find prayer difficult, even meaningless at moments. The Christians who try to encourage and admonish you will irritate you. Their truth about the promise of God is unsettling. ("Why am I in this shape then, if *God is so good*?") You may never say it aloud (and then again, you may) but you will battle immense self-pity, and envy those persons who are doing well. ("Why me and not her?") At those times you will be tempted to distance yourself from the people of God, draw within, and nurse your misfortune. That is when you must press your way to the cover of the House of God.

Most acutely you will be challenged on everything you *ever believed about* God. "If this is not working, then maybe *that too*, was false." In suffering, the enemy comes to unravel the fabric of your spiritual life, so that you will not proceed from faith to FAITH. And he does so primarily, so that you will not survive.

But as for me, my feet had almost slipped. I had nearly lost my foothold. For I envied the arrogant when I saw the prosperity of the wicked. They have no struggles, their bodies are healthy and strong. They are free from the burdens common to man...not plagued by human ills. When I thought to know this it was too painful for me...Until I went into the sanctuary of God. Then I understood...
(Psalm 73:2-5, 16-17 NIV)

Even at fourteen years old, I knew instinctively that I had "better get back to safety," among the saints of God, into the atmosphere of the holy. In the shoot-outs of old western movies, when a person was trying to move to the next place during a gun battle, he always enlisted his allies who were "armed," to cover him.

Even if you have no strength to worship, you need to be among "armed" worshippers.

Even if you cannot recall your own testimony, you need to be within earshot of someone who is reminding you of God's current actions in the earth. They are armed.

Even if in your heart, you are skeptical of

every word the preacher is saying, you need to be positioned to hear it. The atmosphere of the sanctuary becomes a kind of covering while you are fighting to live.

My first week out of the hospital, walking in pain, waiting on the bus alone, I went to the house of God. I was out of ammunition.

In the "sanctified" worship, the time of glorifying God, the time when God was allowed to move freely among the people, I knew my heart was being tested. *What would be the "conditions" on my worship?* Worship collides with the secret attitudes of the heart, and exposes them to you and to the Lord of your praise.

An old sanctified warrior, Mother Mayes, who has long ago gone to heaven, struck up a song. She declared, "Whatever you need, God's got it! Whatever you need, God's got it! He's got everything you need!" The whole church went up in the praise! That day as I danced before the Lord, I danced until the pain left. I danced until the migratory rheumatoid arthritis stopped migrating. THAT DAY I believed in my heart that I was healed.

• Judges and Skeptics

Are there times when you are seated comfortably in your seat of safety? Have you, like David's wife, Michal, judged and even ridiculed those who go forth in abandoned praise? *(II Samuel 6: 14-16)* Does it irritate you, because we take so much time singing to God? Do you think it excessive and unseemly that we shout, run, cry and release ourselves to the Holy Spirit? Do you judge us as merely poor stupid people, overtaken by the mass psychology of the crowd? Sometime we *feel* your tendency to judge us, to ridicule us, and we quench the Spirit who is moving upon us. We put *your* approval above God's welcome.

Little do you know that your skepticism and judgement may be extinguishing some person's <u>very life</u>. Worship opens the door for the entrance of God. Failure to worship shuts the door in His face. Worship breaks the resolve of your enemy to keep coming after you. Worship breaks his will to keep hammering away. *Suffering closes your mouth*, but when you dare to speak out a praise, it *ties up the activity* of the demonic. Worship of the true and living God pushes back principalities arrayed against you, *like a blast of air!*

> *Let the saints be joyful in glory. Let them sing aloud upon their beds [even their sick beds]. Let the high praises of God be in their mouth, and a two-edged sword in their hand…to bind their kings with chains and their nobles with fetters of iron…This honor have all His saints. (Psalm 149: 5-9 KJV)*

Get up right now and raise a praise! Shout to God, dance before Him!! When you sit back down, you will sense the stagnant air around you has moved. Psychiatrists prescribe talking and exercise as adjunct treatments for depression. Talking promotes the release. Physical exercise stimulates you and counteracts the emotional "sludge." The treatment is rooted in the principle of worship. Worship directs your "talk and movement" toward the One who can do something about your condition! Worship breaks the ability of your enemy to remain hunkered down at work in your space. It opens the door to God, and creates an actual sacred space for Him to come and hold court! He can decree the thing you need from that meeting place.

I was waiting on the other side of the door, and I will be eternally grateful for a church family who knew how to "let Him in."

I believed. I received, in the worship encounter with God. Then I confessed it with my mouth. I told the church, I told my friends. I told whom ever would hear. And every time through the years when the enemy brought again the symptoms, *I told the devil*. I knew the work was done! I would not let judges and skeptics keep me from getting what I needed from God. Now I would not let judges and skeptics tell me I didn't have it. Your testimony is your final payment. By it, you overcome!

The first time, I needed the doctor's confirmation. Now I believed, period. I was moving to "big girl" FAITH. *I never saw a doctor again for rheumatoid arthritis.*

Never mistake a 'pop quiz' for a failure. It may only be a refresher of your faith.

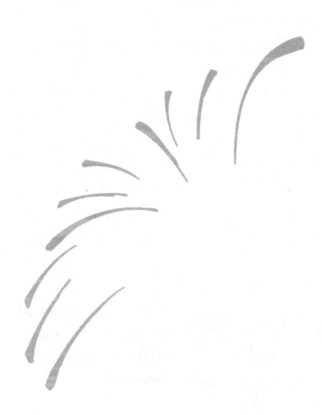

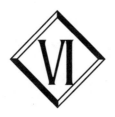

DEVELOPING IN
THE DARKROOM

"When I lay down I say,
'When shall I rise and the night be ended?'
For I have had my fill of tossing till dawn."
(Job 7:4 NKJV)

"Oh my God!" I felt a sick, sinking feeling all over.

"Lord, have mercy!"

It was the last thing that night. The lights were off, the television silenced. Slumber was calling. My husband and I were nestled in for the night. I lazily caressed my breasts to examine them, and my mind stood at attention. I discovered a hard small lump—pronounced, resistant, proud. This was different from the normally dense, spongy matter my breasts were made of. *I was all the way awake.* "David, feel this." I was hoping for assurance from my husband, but yes, he felt it too. Something was different about this.

In the privacy of the next morning, before facing the day, the office, the myriad of counseling needs and administrative functions of our church, I lay in bed savoring a few more moments of solitude. The calm was profound. I looked out at the beauty of the summer trees through my bedroom windows. Then I was jerked again into the moment, like a scampering dog on a short leash. *The lump*. Yes, it was still there. Last night was not an illusion.

I have always been a woman who faces trouble head on. I do not like delays in bad news, evasiveness in relationships, or procrastination in my duty. In characteristic measure, I wanted to face this head on.

I was in my gynecologist's office that very same day. After examination she sought to allay my fears. "You are under 40." "You eat a diet low in fat." "You have no family history of breast cancer." (Only 5% of breast cancers are genetic.) "You do not take hormones or birth control pills." She bundled me up with other assurances and sent me for a mammogram. It was inconclusive. The next step was a sonogram, where the radiologist could look within the breast to the lump itself. The technician looked and looked, long and thoroughly. She then called for the Chief of Radiology to consult with her. In the darkened room, with me on the table, he confidently viewed the scan and assured us both that it was "just a cyst."

"Go home, don't worry. Monitor it. If it bothers you, see your doctor again."

I guess I should thank God that it bothered me.

• **Life Goes On**

For the next six months, the battle was to ascertain whether I was living "by faith" or "in denial." Every girlfriend I trusted, I asked, "Feel this. What do you think?" Meanwhile, I was preaching, teaching, cooking dinner, traveling the evangelistic circuit, entertaining friends, praying for the sick, washing clothes and doing the woman things. Life had to go on. And I was battling this nagging knowing in the corner of my mind, that something terrible just might be gnawing away at my body. I squashed it. I denied it. I pressed beyond it. *I ain't "claiming" nothing negative.* And so I comforted myself.

How many women reading this are living in denial? Editing what you need to say? Censoring what you know? You are trying to outrun your fatigue; your children need you so you just quietly keep going. You deny that you are depressed because you "have to function;" you hush and cry in private. You keep on struggling with a job you hate, a marriage that is killing you, a role you have outgrown — simply because you do not have the courage to face what is true. You have a habit you make excuses for, a secret you will not deal with, because you fear you will lose approval if folks find out.

Or, you have a problem in your body which you will not tend. You say you do not have the money. (Money you would *find* if your child was in trouble.) No time to take off work? (You would *take time* off to sit at the hospital with your mate.) You are "believing God." (But you don't believe *God will accompany* you to the doctor?) Are you living in denial? Could you just be afraid to say you're afraid?

> *...they be many that fight against me, O most High. What time I am afraid, I will trust in Thee. (Psalm 56: 2-3 KJV)*

The lump, like a ticking time bomb, was exponentially dividing and growing. Cancer cells were racing to find tributaries to invade and organs to nestle in, for days of future explosion. Land mines.

After returning from a ministry engagement in December—six months after my sonogram—I confided in my pastoral assistant, Elder Carolyn Ramsey. I was beginning to worry about the pain in my breast. That day, she scheduled an appointment with my surgeon. Before coming into ministry she had been an Oncology Nurse, and was obviously divinely appointed to be in my life at that season.

The next day, my husband and I stopped by the surgeon's office on the way to play a game of tennis. I thought he would perform a routine skinny needle biopsy. A needle would be inserted into the lump, and presuming it was indeed a cyst, fluid would be extracted and examined microscopically.

Indicator number one—he could get no fluid.

My surgeon gave me a prescription for Valium and instructed me to take one before coming into his office the following morning. He would perform a cut-down biopsy on my breast.

The next day, my husband David and my assistant accompanied me to Dr. Richard Fischer's office. I was sedated, numbed, cut and stitched. I waited as his nurse walked my "specimen" across the street to the pathologist. The wait was abnormally long it seemed, but whether it was the calmative effect of the drug or my assurance in God, I presumed I would leave his office and resume life as usual, after this minor inconvenience.

I was terribly wrong.

Most people react in one of two ways when we get bad news. We short out, go blank, go into shock and recall nothing at all. It all becomes a blur. Or, we remember with indelible detail the moment we got life-changing news.

It is as though you are branded with a hot iron. Your child died. You were robbed at gunpoint. You stumbled upon your betrayal. They called with the news of your Daddy's heart attack. The smells of the man who raped you. The sound of metal crashing against your car. The scenes freeze themselves into the walls of your mind.

"Reverend Copeland, there is no good way to give you bad news," Dr. Fischer said as we gathered in his office. I did not want to sit down. "The pathology report shows us a very virulent, aggressive form of cancer. Infiltrating, ductile adenocarcinoma. It is a kind which appears rapidly, grows rapidly and spreads rapidly."

The words bludgeoned me. I was hit between the eyes. My knees buckled under me. My husband and my assistant became dim, distant figures in this surreal conversation that I seemed to be eavesdropping on. Surely he was not talking to me, *about me*. Cancer? My husband and I fumbled through the questions which occurred to us, stumbled home in a daze, and tried to figure out what it was we had just heard.

"Hello, Uncle Thomas? Go over to Mama's house. I've got to tell her some bad news. I don't want her to be alone when she hears." "Hello, Mama. I have cancer." She drops the phone and screams and screams. I think, "I'm glad I called Uncle Thomas." I also think, I am still taking care of everyone else, even at a moment like this.

- ### Ready or Not, Here I Come!

I was just past my thirty-seventh birthday. We had moved into the home of our dreams. My husband had been accepted into a doctoral program at Southern Methodist University. Living, driving and dressing as we chose, giving at the level we had always desired, and we were on an upward spiral in a thriving ministry. I was finding favor, being invited to teach and minister in incredible contexts. I was coming to closure about our infertility, and the probability that I would never bear children, which I so desperately desired. But, I was about to be okay. I was not ready for another fight. Ready or not...

You need to decide about treatment options.

"I opt not to have cancer. Oh well. Too late."

Radical mastectomy or lumpectomy?

"If you only take the lump, what are the chances that you leave some of the cancer?"

If you were my wife, I would strongly advise taking the breast. But of course, it is up to you.

"If you take my entire breast, what are the chances that it has spread to the lymph nodes?"

We'll know after surgery.

"What is chemotherapy going to do to me? How bad will it be?"

Not too bad. We have wonderful drugs to support you and get you through with minimum discomfort.

I don't think he meant to lie.

"What else?"

Because of the position of the lump, radiation would probably permanently injure your lung.

"Skip it."

"Will I lose my hair?"

Yes, probably.

He forgot to mention that he meant <u>everywhere</u>.

"What else?"

Hard to say. The adriamyacin damages the heart. Abrupt menopause. Crushing fatigue. Skin hyper-pigmentation. (Turning ashy-black like a corpse was what he meant.) Mouth sores. Nausea. Vomiting. Not all people react the same way. Regardless. You need the chemotherapy.

"When do we start?"

As soon as possible after the mastectomy.

Oh yeah. Cancer's not bad enough. I need a mastectomy.

Within the week, I was on my way to surgery. The prayer warriors had been alerted, Mama and sister had been summoned, and the congregation had been advised. Ready or not, I was saying goodbye to my breast. The race was on to save my life.

My staff crowded around the door. I awakened with bandages across my chest and tubes draining from my armpit so the lymphatic fluid would not back up into the arm. "How did you cut me?" I feebly asked the doctor. Meaning well, my normally gentle, compassionate physician rebuked me for my superficial concern with vanity. "Oh, don't worry about *that!!* You just get well."

He should have prepared me.

The blackness crowded in upon me until I could scarcely lift my head. *It is getting dark in here.* Tears sat in the reservoir of my belly with no power to reach my eyes. The depression was immobilizing. My husband sat helplessly by my bedside. My assistant became my private nurse, and kept vigil in my room through the night. I was mentally fighting for my life and no outside person could do this for me, but me. The final blow came on the third day.

"I am going to remove the bandages today."

When I saw the horrible bloody snake across my chest, I nearly fainted. The despair smothered me. I was discharged on Christmas Eve 1990, and went home to have a Merry Christmas.

• Snapshots in the Night

PICTURE: Post op week. Renita arrives from Nashville. She is in my house; I hear her footsteps coming up my stairs, stopping outside my bedroom door. I don't want to let her in. Suddenly she's sitting on the side of my bed. "Let me see." I show her, all the while searching her face. She tries to appear unmoved. I know better. She is my friend who has never let me hide from the truth, but never makes me face it alone.

PICTURE: One week after the removal of my breast, I am in the Cayman Islands on a prayer retreat with my preaching sister/friends: Cecelia Williams Bryant, JoAnn Browning, Jessica Kendall Ingram, and me. I cry, I talk. I beg God for courage to go home and face my chemotherapy. They hold me. They cry. They sit in silence with me. They whisper when I am not in the room. We pray. I come home.

PICTURE: A seven-way telephone call the night before my first chemotherapy. All my girlfriends on the line: Renita Weems, Elaine Flake, Barbara Lucas and my Caymen Island sisters. They bathe me in prayer. They hold me up. The doctor has threaded the catheter down my jugular vein, exiting my chest wall, preparing my body to receive what my veins would not tolerate for the next six months. Adriamyacin. 5FU. Cytoxine. That night I feel like a woman preparing for the electric chair. After the first treatment, I rejoice in God. It isn't going to be so bad, after all.

PICTURE: The fourth week after chemotherapy. My hair looks like the hair of a corpse. Wiggy. Dead. Straw-like. I never had much of a figure, not much of a complexion, but I always had hair. Long, luxurious hair. The heritage of my mother's line. My hair has begun to die. I put my "head rag" on tightly at night to secure the remnant of my femininity. When my husband is fast asleep, I tie it under my chin like an old Polish immigrant.

PICTURE: Sitting in the middle of my bathroom floor. Summoning courage. My kitty rubs up against me and just sits and stares, sensing that something is up. In private, I wipe my hands from the forehead back, and take my hair off like a skullcap. I gather it into a plastic bag and stash it under my bathroom sink. Don't ask me why. I call Carolyn, and tell her, dry-eyed. I call my husband, lay in his arms and cry all night long. "Her hair is her glory," they say. Now I get it.

PICTURE: Rummaging through a drawer, looking at the photographic journey of my life. I see a picture of me in a white dress, happy, vibrant and beautiful, preaching and prophesying. So unlike me now. I grab a magic marker and write in a caption *THIS TOO SHALL PASS*. I mount it on my refrigerator door as a prophecy to myself of what shall be, again one day.

PICTURE: At the pulpit. Determined to lift up Jesus. My first Sunday back at New Creation Christian Fellowship after the surgery and the loss of my hair. Strange wig swirling around on my bald head. Tubes still attached to my body, taped down, draining fluid from my under arm. You never know what's beneath those holy preaching robes. The word of the Lord comes forth to the congregation with might and power. *"Let us hold fast the profession of our faith without wavering. Our subject this morning church, is 'Kick But.' Get the 'but' out of your confession, and believe God with a whole heart."* It was a parable on what this ordeal was doing to me. Listeners are often most blessed in the preaching event by eavesdropping on the preacher's worst suffering.

PICTURE: The second month of therapy. David takes me to a Kenneth Copeland meeting at Eagle Mountain, Texas. We are back in the office with Kenneth, Gloria and a young man named Creflo. David requests prayer for me. The Holy Ghost rises in Brother Kenneth and he declares, "I cut the head off this serpent here and now. What you see in days ahead will be just his body in the death throes." I go home that night and pray for every sick woman in my church. The headless serpent is thrashing madly in my mind.

PICTURE: "Claudette, my cancer has resurfaced in the other breast. I go back to surgery this week." My girlfriend Tina, is calling me from New Orleans. We are both in ministry, pastors' wives, sisters in confidence and now in cancer. I go to her bedside. Bald, weakened, I want her to know she's not alone. The devil whispers, "This will be you."

PICTURE: Tina's funeral. Three months after my chemotherapy began. It is kicking my butt. I will never say it publicly. I am seated next to Dr. Betty Price. We are both battling cancer.

When others go to view the body, we both just sit there. At the graveside, I sit in the limousine and clean out my purse.

PICTURE: I am at the pulpit in Milwaukee, Wisconsin preparing to preach. I refuse to stop preaching and giving God glory. I take every engagement I can between treatments. I am reviewing my notes as the choir sings. I feel something wet dripping warmly on my hand. Blood streams down in front of me, from my nose. "Sing another song while I get myself together." *That night, the Holy Ghost sweeps over the church, and mass deliverance takes place. Oh, The Blood...*

PICTURE: After a great Holy Ghost service, my assistant Carolyn and I are back at the hotel room. I place my damp wig on the lamp to dry while we go over the events of the evening and eat our room service meal. I keep saying, "Carolyn, who is pressing hair? I smell hair?" We ignore it and eat our French fries. Later I pick up my wig with a big round light bulb hole in it. I twirl it around on my finger. We crack up laughing. We spend the next day scouting around in the ghetto for a wig store, in a strange town. Gotta be ready for service that night! Some things are funny even on chemotherapy.

PICTURE: I cry in the night. I gaze at my husband's beautiful frame and count the rhythms of his breath while he sleeps. I wonder who he will love after I am dead. I am only halfway through chemotherapy, and I cannot face going back. I tell my doctor I cannot do this. Death would be better. He prescribes anti-anxiety medication so I do not have a panic attack driving to the treatment. I pray in the Spirit. I take my medicine. And I go back.

PICTURE: I'm asleep in bed with my husband. I discern a presence. It is heavy, dark. Someone is in my room. *Someone is in the room with us!!* Standing at the foot of my bed. It is an awful presence. Silent. It starts to lie on me, my feet, my legs. I understand who this is. It is a seducing spirit. Alluring me. "Come and die." I know she wants me to come with her. I am asleep, but in my spirit I shout. I hurl the words, "The blood of Jesus!" And I plead, "Cover me!" She goes away. I tell no one.

PICTURE: I am preaching up a storm at Ray of Hope Christian Church, Atlanta, with my girlfriend, Dr. Cynthia Hale. I am in the middle aisle, in fifth gear. Overdrive! The glory is in the house! The saints are on their feet!! I raise my hands to make a point. "Blooooop." The silicone prosthesis slips out of my bra like a gelatinous mass. In one fluid move, I bend over to stop the rapid descent, somewhere at thigh level. My sister in law, Jackie Copeland, is on the organ. I give her an unexpected cue. "Hit that organ, girl! I feel a praise coming on!" PRAISE HIM EVERYBODY. I run, bent over, back to the platform. I crouch behind Dr. Hale's wooden pulpit. I maneuver under my robes with the skill of a magician and re-plop the prosthesis into place. I reappear and ask the congregation, "Now where was I?" *I have gotten away!*

After the benediction, Mother Mary Ellen Goodwin makes a beeline to greet me at the altar. In an incredulous, *loud* voice she asks, "Did I just see you lose your bosom?" *Shoot!*

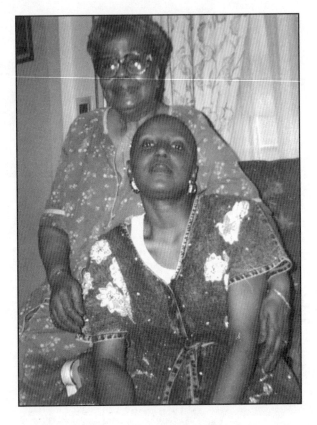

PICTURE: I want my Mama. She calls me. She prays. But I need to see her face. Sit at her kitchen table. I shuffle off to Buffalo. She cooks me collard greens and sweet potatoes and tries to make me eat. I lay my bald head on her. We go to her Baptist church on Sunday morning. For the first time in our adult life, she takes me by the hand and leads _me_ to the altar for prayer. Every preaching woman needs a Mama.

PICTURE: I am sitting in my living room with my best and dearest girlfriend. My discernment still works. The Holy Ghost says, "Danger!!" I want to silence Him. I suddenly realize I need all my energy to fight for my life. I have no time to look over my shoulders at her, and her boundaries in my home. *Eject now. Ask questions later*. In these times when your walls are broken down, the enemy takes liberties.

PICTURE: I am curled up in the fetal position. Hooked to my intravenous pouch of adria. It is my at-home chemo-bag. I am wiped out. I wake up. Wet. The tube has broken. Contamination. Medicinal poison is all over my body, my bedclothes, my mattress. My husband is away preaching. Mama lives 2,000 miles away. I have no child. I must call on Carolyn (again) and I am so embarrassed to keep asking for help. I climb down and just lay on the floor. *Lord, have mercy.* I roll over and put on a tape. Reverend Jackie McCullough of New York preaching "Coming Out of the Stink." Noah in the ark. This stinks. This stinks.

PICTURE: Blinds are closed. Door is shut. I

am not answering the phone. I've just preached two nights. It's taking longer and longer to get my "virtue" back. I am distancing myself from the saints. They call to encourage me and then they ambush. ("You know my Aunt Bessie had what you have. She did well on her chemo and radiation. Real good! Of course her cancer came back five years later, and she died.") Ambushed! Get off my phone! I open my mail. It is a tape from Mother Ruvader Hall, South Bend, Indiana. It is a message I have preached. Something about victory or praise or ...whatever. I am enraged.

Eat your words, Claudette.

Thank God, my words were God's Words.

Thank God, for the Mothers of the Church.

PICTURE: I am puttering around my bedroom closet late one night. Bald. Barely able to climb above the fatigue. Thinking about "what if?" *I am feeling weepy.* What would I give to my sister Stacy, to Mama, to Carolyn, to my 'play daughter' Antonette? My 5-year-old God-daughter Crystal Nicole is playing with her toys on my floor before bedtime. She begins to sing a song I do not know.

Don't cry for me
Don't shed a tear.
The time I shared with you will always be
And when I'm gone
Please carry on
Don't cry for me.

Don't cry for me, when life is not the joy it
should be
With life comes pain
Soon time will end its course appointed
And you'll be rewarded
And all the world will see…
Don't cry for me.
(BeBe and CeCe Winans[1])

She climbs up into bed with me. She rubs
my bald head with one hand and sucks her
thumb on the other. "I love you, Big Mama."
"I love you too, sweet baby."
Skip the self-pity, Claudette. Life is worth
living. I decide to keep my clothes.

PICTURE: It is the eighth month of
chemotherapy. It was only supposed to last
for six. My blood count has not recovered. I

---

[1]Written by B. Winans and K. Thomas for Yellow Elephant
Music, Inc. HEAVEN, Capitol Music, Inc. 1988.

am totally bald. I am black, hyper-pigmented all over. My fingernails and toenails are black. I have sores in my mouth, and other mucous membranes. The smells, foods and activities I enjoyed almost all make me sick. I feel like I have lead in every cell of my body. I am standing naked in my bathroom as I step out of my shower. I see a half-dead woman in the mirror, a snake scar across a vacant chest, catheter dangling from the other side. I am feeling dissociated from my body, barely connected to life.

Suddenly the contradiction explodes in my mind. Indignation rises from some deep place in my soul. I AM NOT GOING OUT LIKE THIS! I feel like the Incredible Hulk or Clark Kent, coming out of the telephone booth. I tap into the spirit realm. *Whether in the body or not, I wonder?* I see the principalities hovering, waiting like vultures to take me out. The Greater One arises within me!! I speak directly to the Evil One. His foul presence hangs in my atmosphere. Like a runner, from out of nowhere I have "second wind." I have broken through the wall of terror. I am not intimidated. I am not afraid. I have nothing to lose.

"DEVIL, YOU BETTER KILL ME IF YOU CAN. KILL ME WHILE I AM DOWN, IF YOU CAN. BECAUSE WHEN I GET UP FROM THIS, I AM COMING BACK WITH POWER. I WILL BE ARMED, AND EXCEEDINGLY DANGEROUS."

That moment I know. He cannot. He wants to. He aimed to. He tried to… but He has no authority to take my life. That night God gives me Isaiah 41:15, a text I do not know.

I will make thee a new sharp threshing instrument, having teeth, and thou shall thresh the mountains, and beat them small.

PICTURE: I am off chemotherapy. My hair is coming back like silky peach fuzz. I venture out in public for the first time without my wig. I have on makeup and earrings, on my way to a preaching engagement. I think I am pretty cute for the first time in a year. My husband drops me off at the curb of the airport. I am standing tall. I feel new life budding. I check my bags curbside. I smile. I feel people staring. I feel eyes on the back of my head. I look at them and they look away. I see a little kid pointing at my head. My confidence is fading fast. I hand the gate agent my ticket and he averts his gaze. No one will look at me. My presence makes them too uncomfortable. By the time I get to my seat on the plane, I pull out my head rag and wrap my head.

That's okay, though.

Tomorrow is another day. And I *am planning* to have a tomorrow!!

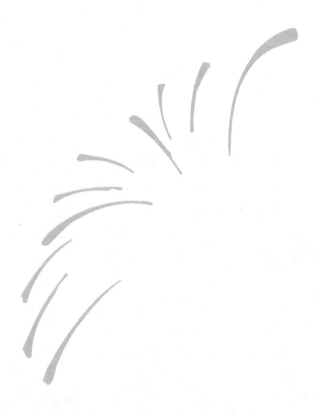

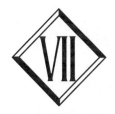

THE DAYSTAR ARISES

"We also have a more sure word of prophecy, whereunto you do well that you take heed. As a light that shines in a dark place, until the day dawn, and the Daystar arise in your heart." (II Peter 1:19 KJV)

All suffering is disorienting. The journey back to wholeness can be tricky. Recovering from a divorce and believing you will ever be happy again, seems improbable. Healing your heart from the death of your child, your parent, your love, may seem impossible. So much is shattered. You have no sense of where to even begin. Likewise, coming out of cancer is like coming out of darkness. It is done respectfully, tentatively. And it is a step-by-step process. The darkness is so overwhelming, you strain to find your bearings. You peer into the horizon for flickers of light. But once you find a point of light, fasten your eyes on it, and do not let it out of your sight.

When you face the most terrorizing life-threatening medical procedures, keep your eyes upon the Light. When you must fight with insurance companies about what you know is necessary but they say is "cosmetic," (then they drop you anyway rather than pay the bills) look straight up. When you go back for the bone scan because you have stray pains that just might be cancer, you must fasten on the Light. When you are haunted by symptoms; when your liver function tests are off; when your friends have recurrences and die; you fasten on the Light. Even though the darkness surrounds you, God locates you. He has not lost nor misplaced you.

> *If I say, surely the darkness shall cover me, even the night shall be light about me. Yea, the darkness hides not from Thee, but the night shines as the day. Darkness and light are both alike to Thee. (Psalm 139:11-12 KJV)*

You must not allow suffering to make you *lose Him*.

This Light is not a metaphysical concept. Not

a meditative practice. It is the presence of God as your gift. *"Light is sown for the righteous," says Psalm 97:11.* When darkness is so thick "it may be felt," God's children have light in their dwelling. *(Exodus 10:21-23).* It pays to learn the Light, to recognize Him and walk in Light, before the darkness hits.

- **Trust**

The darkness makes us tap within. It makes us consult the map of memory. Darkness takes away all the devices of our flesh which once served us – rods, corneas, retinas. None of the human tools can work without external light to aid them. We must trust the internal deposit of God. We gravitate to the "territory of experience" with God— or we urgently seek to have one. We seek our solutions in His mystery. Darkness teaches you to ***trust what you already know.***

I travel often and lodge in unfamiliar hotel rooms. In the rush to meet a service time or in the post preaching fatigue, I am guilty of leaving the room in disarray. A suitcase on the floor and shoes or books where they land. Then comes night. I am too tired to rearrange things, too weary to straighten up. I go to bed. But I have begun the practice of leaving a light on in the bathroom, and closing the door.

I will inevitably need to 'go' several times during the night.

In spite of the obstacles, the clutter of shoes and books, the suitcase in the middle of the floor, and the disarray of an unfamiliar room, the journey through the darkness is mandatory. I will have to go to the bathroom. It matters not that I am dead tired and disoriented. It is irrelevant that I don't remember the hotel name, or the room number, and sometime not even the city I am in. I can no longer lay there in the darkness. The urge makes me get up. I have to go. Then I remember. I have a point of light in the dark room. I know where I am trying to go.

It is dark around your life. Tonight you think you will never feel good again. But don't just lay there. You have to get up. *Don't you feel the urge?* Tonight you are disheartened by the image in the mirror, all your beauty faded away. Tonight, pain makes you believe that death would be preferable to this. Tonight you see pity or superficial gaiety in the eyes of your friends. You sense distance in the heart of your lover and you wonder if you will ever be desirable again. You are disoriented because your companion is gone and your money has dried up and you do not have a clue about what to do with the rest of your wretched, pitiful life. But don't lay there in the dark.

Respect the inner urge to *go. Then get up.*

I get up. I see the sliver of light under the bathroom door. I trip. I stumble. I hit my shins and my toes in the dark. I hurt myself at times. But I can't stop going where I need to be. Just beyond the door is the place I will lay my burden down, release the stuff I need not hold. Just beyond the door is a flood of light.

Trust the light. Keep moving toward it. With outstretched hands, feel your way.

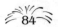

You are almost at the doorknob.

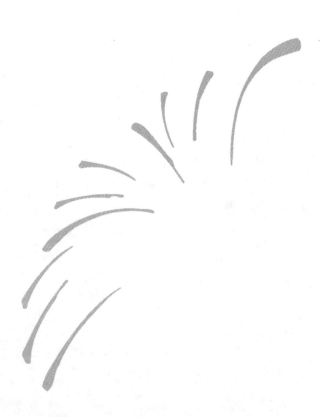

EPILOGUE:
IF I SHOULD
DIE BEFORE I
WAKE

Now I lay me down to sleep
I pray Thee Lord my soul to keep
If I should die before I wake
I pray Thee Lord my soul to take.

It has been ten years since my cancer diagnosis. At the ninth year out, something appeared in my remaining breast. That old familiar season of horror rolled up on the screen, like a bad re-run.

I have seen this before. It was <u>not</u> a good movie.

I opted for a lumpectomy. It was benign.

Pop Quiz.

There are those reading this whose story ends differently. Some of you are not getting well. You love God. You have persevered in faith. You have done all you know, spiritually and medically. And yet, you cannot deny it. You are dissolving. **Your healing will be in your exit from this body.** Your spirit is turning, less invested now, in all that has been. You are dying. And you wish on some level, that you could talk about it.

This epilogue is for you.

Gently, respectfully, let me sit by your side. Lay your head upon my lap. Let me lie next to you in your bed. Allow me to speak into your ear.

Most Christian sisters and brothers will <u>not</u> know how to speak with you of death or dying. Most have never even looked long in this direction, much less, ventured close to the edge of life. They will not know how to listen to you. Too awkward. Too paralyzed. Too puzzled. Not wanting to see what they see.

Do not be too surprised or offended if they

disappear. "I just don't know what to say."
They drift away one by one, melding back into
the woodwork of their lives, their church,
their work, their days. The Christians will be
silent because they are trying to make you
comfortable, but mainly because they
themselves are so uncomfortable. Your dying
reminds them. They see in you a dress
rehearsal for themselves.

Preachers are the custodians of spiritual
things, but we may also come short of your
hopes. We will insist that you "keep a positive
attitude." "Hold on to hope." We will toss
you some worn clichés, or some favorite
scriptures that are not even *your* favorites.
Or we will cut directly to the "let me pray for
you" mode. You tolerate our prayers. You
would rather have had a genuine nourishing
conversation.

Most of your family will "hush" you. If you
desire to speak freely of your business affairs,
your Will, where to find your insurance
papers; how you want your funeral service;
they will say, "Hush now." If you ask to talk,

<u>really</u> talk about some unfinished business, ask forgiveness, start saying goodbye—you will send them scurrying behind phrases. "Don't talk like that!" And it shuts you down.

Try not to die lonely.

- **Night Vision**

The prospect of your dying is terrorizing for your family and friends because they are losing you. The reality of dying is harder on you, because you are *losing them, and everything else surrounding this life*.

Love is strong as death, says scripture. "Because at the hour of a man's death the parting of the soul and body is difficult; because there is no love, no attachment, no mixture like that of soul and body." And jealousy is cruel as the grave. "...There is no jealousy in the world like that of the [woman] who goes to her grave and sees that the world still lives." So wrote 18th century rabbi Elijah ben Shlomo Zalman. And so it is today.

Dying pries away your dreams of what might

have been. You are losing what you had expected to witness, experience, and to enjoy. Dying is a robbery of all things. It is drawing you through portals of anger and depression and even momentarily, to despair. Paul labels it the last enemy which shall be destroyed. (I Corinthians 15:26). If we are not wise and sober, even the prospect of dying can rob us of the good days we have till then.

Now is the time to discover that you have everything to gain.

As we have born the image of the man of dust, we shall also bear the image of the heavenly Man. Now I say this brethren, that flesh and blood cannot inherit the kingdom of God, nor does corruption inherit incorruption. (vv. 49-50 NKJV)

But first, you must drop off this body. In legal terms, some things are received pro bono, *free of charge, by the goodness of another*. Others are received quid pro quo, *something in exchange for something*. The life-death-life transaction is both. The price which makes *us deserving* of Heaven was the death of God's son; we receive eternal life freely by grace. Yet the passage to *enter* is "something in exchange for something." We must die in order to live. We must drop off this dissolving, wasting body to inherit one which will stand up outside of time, throughout all eternity. This next step is quid pro quo. Today on this side, the exchange seems so uneven, so unjust. You never want to release what you know, for that which cannot be seen.

Unless of course, you get night vision. Night vision *takes the terror out of dying*, for we have gotten a revelation of what–and Who—awaits on the other side.

So we fix our eyes, not on that which is seen, but on what is unseen. For what is seen is temporary, but what is unseen is eternal. (II Corinthians 4:18 NIV)

I have a kitty. For her own reasons, she will wait till the lights are out and everyone is in bed, to play. She will romp, scamper, jump, leap and bound all over my house. And she never lets furniture be an obstacle nor does she collide with the fixtures. She sees them in the dark. Or maybe she senses things with internal radar. Or navigates with an inate map.

She has night vision. I think maybe we all have it. We just do not tap in.

Night vision stops you from colliding head on, with despair. It diverts you, sliding toward depression head on, and leads you out. It alerts you to the whispers of suicide in the dark and turns your heart. Night vision guards you from tumbling headlong into stupid sexual choices or unlawful emotional liaisons—*counterfeit comfort* while you are going through. Night vision is necessary you see, to sense eternity.

Now it is God who has made us for this purpose [eternity] And has given us the Spirit as a deposit, guaranteeing what is to come! (II Corinthians 5:5 NIV)

Paul declares that while we are in this tent, "we groan and are burdened because we do not want to be unclothed." We dread stepping out of this body. But we "do wish to be clothed with our heavenly dwelling so that what is mortal may be swallowed up by Life." Night vision sees beyond this present darkness, the present condition, into the land of perfect day. Night vision sees HIM

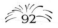

who comes Himself, to take the sting out of death, and the victory out of the grave.

The conversation with Him whom your night vision discerns, shall be the sweetest ever upon your tongue.

"Abide with me, fast falls the eventide. The darkness deepens, Lord with me abide;
When other helpers fail and comforts flee, Helper of the helpless, O abide with me.

Swift to its close ebbs out life's little day; Earth's joys grow dim, its glories pass away.
Change and decay in all around I see; O thou who changest not, abide with me.

I need Thy presence every passing hour; What but Thy grace can foil the tempter's power?
Who like Thyself, my guide and stay can be? Through cloud and sunshine, O abide with me.

I fear no foe with Thee at hand to bless. Ills have no weight and tears no bitterness.
Where is death's sting? Where grave Thy

victory? I triumph still if Thou abide with me.

Hold thou Thy cross before my closing eyes. *Shine through the gloom, and point me to the skies.*

Heaven's morning breaks, and earth's vain shadows flee. In life, in death. O Lord, abide with me."[2]

Long for Him. Look for Him through this dark night of the soul. See Him who comes again for you. He alone abides, and He alone is enough.

• **Before I Die...**

One final thing. If you should die, *before* you die, take control of your life in the time you have! In whatever way you choose, whatever way you are able, redeem the days that remain. Well-meaning family and friends may take decisions out of your hands presuming to lighten your load. They may tell you what "is best" for you, never having a clue where you really are. They may walk a wide circle around you, ignoring your basic needs to be touched, hugged, and held. They think you're too fragile. They are afraid they

---

[2]Henry F. Lyte, "Abide With Me", *Pilgrim Hymnal* (Boston: Pilgrim Press, 1958)

will "catch" what you have. They may say you "need your rest" while they are really backing away, preparing <u>themselves</u> for the time they'll be without you.

OPEN YOUR EYES. OPEN YOUR MOUTH! OPEN YOURSELF TO THE WONDER THAT IS YOURS THIS DAY. Put your fingerprints on the environment! Seize the day! Tell them your wishes! You *may be* dying. Frankly, we all are, whether sick or well, old or young. BUT YOU ARE NOT DEAD TODAY!

And you still have wishes and needs and options. You still have the option to receive Christ if you have not. He is your passport and your guide through the turbulent waters of death, and into the presence of the Father. Ask Him today to come in, to forgive you, to save you, and believe that He has. It is never too late to tend to the business of your soul. Open your mouth and say something! Say it to God. And say it to the persons who matter.

◇ Tell them to roll your bed over by the window, even if you're too weak to get out of it.

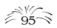

◇ Write those letters.

◇ Take that trip you keep putting off. <u>Some-one</u> will travel with you.

◇ Walk through the mall…at your own pace.

◇ Spray on some perfume at the cosmetic counter.

◇ Take a class. Then take another one.

◇ Pick up the telephone and <u>tell</u> her, "I miss you. Come and see me."

◇ Reach out and hold his hand. You need to be touched. Touch.

◇ Laugh, laugh, laugh. It's medicine. A lot of stuff is still funny.

◇ Eat what you love…even if you can only eat a little of it now.

◇ Forgive them. Let them go.

◇ Tell the physicians you appreciate all they are doing for you. But now you want to make another decision about your treatment, your medication, your body.

◇ Forgive God.

◇ You fill in the blank.

"If I should die before I wake…"

This was the first prayer I ever learned as a child. A journey through thick darkness and prolonged nights, *illuminated* the power in this prayer.

If I should die before I wake, may I make good decisions about the days I have left. If I should die before I wake, let me suck the marrow out of life 'til it is dry-white, like the neck-bones I ate as a child. May I live life like it is going out of style!!!

◇ Let me nuzzle and kiss the neck folds of a tiny baby while she sleeps.

◇ Let me scoop warm sand with pedicured toes, as salty Caribbean water washes over my legs.

◇ Let me smell the freshly cut summer grass, one more season.

◇ Let me give extravagant gifts to my friends, and watch their hearts smile.

◇ Let a young man glance at me, just once more, with lingering appreciation in his eyes. And let me glance back, with a twinkle in mine.

◇ Let me walk hand in hand with my sister up the street from Mama's house, in the Fall when the leaves turn red and orange and gold, and let me watch her children play.

◇ Let me spy from my window, the world at rest, asleep, snug under blankets of freshly fallen snow. Then let me startle it with my frolic and footprints in remembrance of youthful days and innocent dreams till the nostalgia hurts my heart, then makes me bow in humble gratitude.

◇ Let me make wild, wet, abandoned love, nourished by the skin and sinews, smell and soul of my beloved. Just one more time.

◇ Let me empty my thoughts, risk my secrets, deposit my lessons into someone's life who will be wise enough to use them after I am gone.

And let me die, while I still love God.

And he showed me a pure river of

Water of life

Clear as crystal, proceeding out of the throne of

God and of the Lamb.

In the midst of the street of it,

And

On either side of the river was there,

The Tree of Life...

And the leaves of the tree were for the healing of

The nations

And his servants shall serve Him

And they shall see His face...

And there shall be no night there...

For the Lord giveth them light.

Revelation 22: 1-5

THOUGHTS, PRAYERS, DECISIONS

ABOUT THE AUTHOR

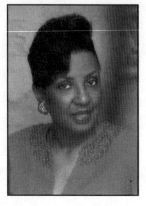 THE REVEREND DR. CLAUDETTE A. COPELAND presently serves as Pastor and Co-Founder of the New Creation Christian Fellowship Church of San Antonio, Texas. Dr. Copeland has a profound sensitivity to the suffering of young people as a survivor of repeated childhood illnesses. Diagnosed with breast cancer in 1990, she found God leading her to make use of her suffering in tangible ways.

She entered a Doctor of Ministry preaching cluster and designed a program that reached beyond the pulpit, to explore the interior regions of grief and loss in the life of believers. Her doctoral thesis, *Developing A Model for Ministering To Grief and Loss In The Local Church Congregation: A Study in Transformation* was forged as she completed cancer treatment.

Dr. Copeland is a former Military Chaplain (U.S.A.F.), Hospital Chaplain, and is a member of the Association for Clinical Pastoral Education. She is a former Mentor for doctoral studies and Visiting Professor at United Theological Seminary, Dayton, Ohio. She is a sought after lecturer, workshop leader and preacher in cross-denominational circles, nationally and internationally. She was featured by Ebony Magazine as one of the 15 Great African American Women Preachers, and is included in the Smithsonian Institute (Anacostia Museum) "Speak To My Heart" Exhibit: Communities of Faith and Contemporary African American Lives.

She is married to the Bishop David Michael Copeland, Senior Pastor of New Creation Christian Fellowship and Prelate of The Kingdom Council of Interdependent Christian Churches and Ministries. They reside in San Antonio, Texas.

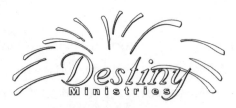
Destiny
Ministries

**Other Products By
The Reverend Dr. Claudette A.
Copeland
May be obtained by contacting
Destiny Ministries
12521 Nacogdoches Road,
San Antonio, Texas 78217
210-646-7997 Extension 214
Or visit us on-line at**
www.ClaudetteACopeland.org

Audio Tape Series Include

*Christians With an Attitude
(The Issue of Offenses)
Woman Wisdom
(Training Godly Women)
Fighting for the Family
Walk In the Spirit
(An Exposition of Galatians 5:19-21)
The Secret Storms
(Real Life Woman-Dilemmas)
Sex and Sexuality
(Perspectives for Christian Women)
Conceive and Bring Forth
(Birthing Spiritual Realities)
The Revelation of Wealth
(Having and Handling Money)
...and more!*
*
*Music Compact Disc
"Altogether Lovely, My Beloved" With Sister
Renetha
(An exquisite experience in worship)*